I0441295

LOW FODMAP

LOW-FODMAP DIET COOKBOOK –

80 EASY AND DELICIOUS GASTROINTESTINAL-FRIENDLY RECIPES

TO COMFORT YOUR DIGESTIVE DISORDERS

(THE IBS, QUIET GUT, ULCERATIVE COLITIS, CROHN'S DISEASE COOKBOOK)

Complete Authorized Edition

BY

MARY CRISWELL-CARPENTER

© **Copyright 2016 by Mary Criswell-Carpenter- All rights reserved.**

In any way it is illegal to reproduce, duplicate, or transmit any part of this document in either electronic means or in printed format. Recording of this publication is strictly prohibited and any storage of this document is not allowed unless with written permission from the publisher. All rights reserved.

The information provided herein is stated to be truthful and consistent, in that any liability, in terms of inattention or otherwise, by any usage or abuse of any policies, processes, or directions contained within is the solitary and utter responsibility of the recipient reader. Under no circumstances will any legal responsibility or blame be held against the publisher for any reparation, damages, or monetary loss due to the information herein, either directly or indirectly.

Respective authors own all copyrights not held by the publisher.

Legal Notice:

This book is copyright protected. This is only for personal use. You cannot amend, distribute, sell, use, quote or paraphrase any part or the content within this book without the consent of the author or copyright owner. Legal action will be pursued if this is breached.

Disclaimer Notice:

Please note the information contained within this document is for educational and entertainment purposes only. Every attempt has been made to provide accurate, up to date and reliable complete information. No warranties of any kind are expressed or implied. Readers acknowledge that the author is not engaging in the rendering of legal, financial, medical or professional advice.

By reading this document, the reader agrees that under no circumstances are we responsible for any losses, direct or indirect, which are incurred as a result of the use of information contained within this document, including, but not limited to, —errors, omissions, or inaccuracies.

Table of Contents

Oat Encrusted Fish with Salad of Baby Greens (4 Servings)

Pad Thai Noodles (4 Servings)

Parmesan Coated Wings (24 Servings)

Pineapple Bites (4 Servings)

Potato Salad (5 Servings)

Quinoa and Cucumber Salad (4 Servings)

Quinoa with Almonds and Feta Salad (4 Servings)

Raspberry-Coconut Bars (16 Servings)

Rice and Tuna Salad (4 Servings)

Salad Niçoise (4 Servings)

Savory Chicken and Rice Muffins (8 Servings)

Smoked Salmon Appetizers (20 Servings)

Spinach and Butternut Squash Salad (6 Servings)

Spring Soup (4 servings for an appetizer, 2 for dinner)

Tuesday Tacos (4 Servings)

Turkey Burgers with Spinach and Feta (4 Servings)

Chapter 4:   Low-FODMAP Dinner Recipes

Bacon Wrapped Chicken Thighs with Spicy Rice (4 Servings)

Baked Tilapia with Roasted Vegetable Assortment (2 Servings)

Beef Tips in Red Wine Sauce (4 Servings)

California Sushi Rolls (12 Servings)

Cheesy Spinach and Quinoa (4 Servings)

Chicken and Tomatoes in Cream Sauce (4 Servings)

Chinese Eggplant (3 Servings)

Classic Roast Beef with Vegetables (6 Servings)

Fried Rice (4 Servings)

Gingery Egg Drop Soup (4 Servings)

Greek Chicken (6 Servings)

Lemon-Herb Topped Tilapia with Baby Greens and Basmati Rice (4 Servings)

Lemon Pepper Chicken and Rice (4 Servings)

New Potato Salad with Green Beans and Anchovies (1 Serving)

Roasted Leg of Lamb (6 Servings)

Shepherd's Pie (4 Servings)

Shrimp Scampi (4 Servings)

Almond Cake with Fruit Compote (10 Servings)

Blueberry Coconut Ice Cream (1 Liter)

Brie with Raspberry Compote (4 Servings)

Choco-Chia Peanut Butter Pudding (2 Servings)

Chocolate Cobbler 6 Servings

Crunchy Chocolate and Raspberry Parfait (4 Servings)

Fudge Pie with Raspberries (12 Servings)

Fudgy Rich Brownies (12 Servings)

Lemon Coconut Cookies (14 Servings)

Pecan Sandies (22 Servings)

Pumpkin Pie Filling (8 Servings)

Orange Cranberry Pudding (7 Servings)

Rhubarb Parfait (6 Servings)

Rice Pudding (4 Servings)

Strawberries in the Clouds (4 Servings)

Strawberry Crumble (4 Servings)

Introduction

I want to thank you and congratulate you for downloading the book, **Low FODMAP: 80 Easy and Delicious Gastrointestinal-Friendly Recipes to Comfort your Digestive Disorders.** This revision is the complete authorized edition, published to replace **Low FODMAP: 77 Easy and Delicious Gastrointestinal-Friendly Recipes to Comfort your Digestive Disorders**.

This book contains proven steps and strategies on why eating low-FODMAP foods are best for a nutritional food program for people with IBS, Crohn's Disease, Ulcerative Colitis, and other disorders. It is chock-full of enticing, easy recipes that you can eat properly with a busy weekday schedule.

Eating low-FODMAP encourages a lifestyle change, not a temporary fix to your IBS or digestive disorder dilemma. Choosing a healthy eating plan will enhance your energy and invigorate your health. When you follow the suggested recipes, eating at the proper times, you will have a much easier time dealing with the discomforts of your digestive disorder

Thanks again for downloading this book, I hope you enjoy it!

Chapter 1: .. How and Why a Low FODMAP Diet Will Help You with Your IBS

To begin with understanding why a low FODMAP Diet would be helpful in your personal circumstance, let us begin with what a FODMAP might be. A FODMAP is an abbreviation for a collection of short-chain carbohydrates found in many everyday table foods. FODMAPs stands for Fermentable Oligo-, Di- and Mono-saccharides, and Polyols.

Doctors at Monash University, in Australia, have iniatated a new approach for Irritable Bowel Syndrome and similar digestive disorders treatment. This approach is one that involves patients voluntarily following a low-FODMAP diet as a way to decrease and sometimes totally halt aggravating and debilitating IBS symptoms.

Those scientists have promoted the FODMAP theory, that is consuming foods that are high in FODMAPS will increase the pain and reduce the motility of foods in the large and small intestine. As these foods slow down in the digestive system they produce the predictable symptoms of IBS, such as abdominal pain, bloating, diarrhea, gas and constipation.

These doctors propose that following their low-FODMAP diet will lessen and even eliminate the awful unexpected attacks of Irritable Bowel Syndrome, Crohn's Disease, and Ulcerative Colitis. They have documented success in over 70% of the persons that faithfully follow this plan.

One of the theories of the Australian doctors' is that there is a cumulative effect of high FODMAP foods on the digestive system. If you eat the high FODMAP foods as a regular diet, you will have more drastic and debilitating symptoms than you would if you only ate one food for a limited time.

People with IBS, Crohn's Disease, and Ulcerative Colitis have found they have sensitivities to many foods and the FODMAP Diet addresses the most common trigger foods. You will find the need to add your own personal lists as you develop the information.

This book has recipes that are suggested for the FODMAP Diet. It does not substitute for a medical staff and dietitian for your diagnosis and treatment plan. You may be tempted to follow only part of the diet, or conversely, hurriedly go into a diet that is developed to be attempted in stages. Working with your personal medical team will be the best way to ensure your continued progressing good health.

Chapter 2 Low FODMAP Breakfast Recipes

Apple and Linseed Oatmeal (4 Servings)

Per Serving = Calories: 56 – Fat:6 g – Carbs:29 g – Protein:12 g

Ingredients:

- 100g porridge oats
- 2 eating apples, peeled and grated
- ½ tsp ground cinnamon, plus extra for sprinkling
- 500ml skimmed milk
- 2 tbsp ground linseed
- 150ml pot probiotic yogurt
- drizzle of honey

Directions:

On a medium flame, mix the first four ingredients, oats, apples, cinnamon and almond milk (if you are lactose intolerant) in a saucepan. Bring to a boil while stirring, then turn to a low flame and cook an additional 5 minutes, whilst continuing to stir.

Add the ground linseeds, then divide to serve in 4 bowls for the table. Each bowl can be topped with a spoon of yogurt and honey, and a sprinkle or two of cinnamon. Nutmeg is also good for a sprinkle.

Bacon and Brie Frittata (4 Servings)

Per Serving = Calories: 395 – Fat:31 g – Carbs:3 g – Protein:25 g

Ingredients:

- 2 T olive oil
- 200g smoked bacon
- 6 egg
- lightly beaten
- small bunch chives, snipped
- 100g brie, sliced
- 1 tsp red wine vinegar
- 1 tsp Dijon mustard
- 1 cucumber, halved, deseeded and sliced on the diagonal
- 200g radish, quartered

Directions:

Heat 1 teaspoon of oil in a small skillet that is not-stick. Add the bacon and fry until crispy. Place on a paper towel to drain while you do the next step.

Heat 2 teaspoons of oil into the same frying pan. Crumble the bacon, add the eggs, chives and black pepper and cook until the eggs are partially set. Now lay the Brie cheese on top. Grill until the eggs are set. Remove the omelette from the pan and cut into 8 wedges, placing 2 on each plate.

Mix a salad of the olive oil, vinegar, mustard, seasonings, cucumbers and radishes together and stir to thoroughly saturate the mixture. Place on the plate between the two omelette wedges.

Baked Eggs and Ham Cups (4 servings)

Per Serving = Calories: 520 – Fat: 7g – Carbs: 1g – Protein: 14g

Ingredients:

- 8 Slices of ham
- 2 T grated parmesan cheese
- 4 whole eggs
- 150g of baby spinach
- 4 slices of buttered toast

Directions:

Begin by preheating your oven to 350F degrees. Grease four different oven-safe dishes that can hold ¾ cup, like ramekins. Place 2 slices of ham in each dish, covering the bottom and sides.

Microwave your spinach for a minute and a half, then drain it in a colander, pushing and pressing the spinach to remove all excess water.

Divide the spinach as evenly as possible between the ramekins, atop the ham slices. Place 2 T of parmesan cheese on the spinach.

Break the eggs, one at a time, over each dish gently, so as not to break the yolk. Salt and pepper to taste.

Place all the ramekins on one baking tray and place in the oven for fifteen minutes. Bake until the yolks are set to your desired doneness.

Banana Blast (serves 1)

Per Serving = Calories: 272 – Fat:8 g – Carbs: 45 g – Protein: 8 g

Ingredients:

1 banana

1 T oats

1 T flaxseed

1 T cinnamon

1 cup almond milk

1 tsp coconut flavoring

1 ice cube

Directions:

Combine all ingredients into a blender and blend until thick and creamy.

Enjoy!

Buckwheat Groat Bread with Seeded Topping (8 Servings)

Per Serving = Calories: 310 – Fat:17 g – Carbs: 34g – Protein: 4g

Ingredients:

- 1 1/2 cups gluten-free plain flour
- 1/2 cup buckwheat flour
- 3 teaspoons gluten-free baking powder
- 1/2 teaspoon Pink Himalayan Salt Flakes
- 2 tablespoons superfine sugar
- 2 egg whites, warmed to room temperature
- 1 cup reduced-fat milk
- 1/2 cup vegetable oil
- 2 tablespoons seed mix with pine nuts

Directions:

Preheat oven to 350F. Line with parchment paper and then grease a 9 x 5 inch loaf pan.

Sift the flour, baking powder and salt into a large, pourable bowl. Add the sugar and mix carefully.

Place the egg whites in a warmer bowl (not cold, but not heated) and beat the egg whites until they are just frothy. Stir in the milk and oil and continue to beat. Add this mixture to the flour mix and beat for 2 or 3 minutes, until the lumps are gone and the mixture is smooth.

Pour the mixture into the prepared loaf pan. Smooth the top with a spatula to make it evenly spread in the pan. Press the seed mix lightly into mixture. Bake for 55 minutes to 1 hour or until a knife inserted in the center of the bread comes out clean. Leave the bread to cool in the pan for 10 minutes. Flip bread onto a towel in your hand, then upright onto a wire rack to cool.

Carrot Cake with Pecans (8 Servings)

Per Serving = Calories: 599 – Fat:28 g – Carbs:86 g – Protein:6 g

Ingredients:

- 140g unsalted butter, softened, plus extra for greasing
- 200g caster sugar
- 250g carrots, grated
- 140g sultanas
- 2 eggs, lightly beaten
- 200g gluten-free self-rising flour
- 1 tsp cinnamon
- 1 tsp gluten-free baking powder
- 50g pecans, chopped

For the icing

- 75g butter, softened
- 175g icing sugar
- 3 tsp cinnamon plus extra for dusting

Directions:

Heat oven to 350F. Grease and line a 2 lb bread loaf pan with baking parchment.

Beat the butter and sugar with a mixer until soft and fluffy, then add the grated carrot and sultanas. Add the eggs into the mixing bowl one at a time, scraping and stirring after each addition.

Add the flour, cinnamon, baking powder and most of the chopped pecans and mix well. Pour the mix into the loaf tin, then bake for 50-55 mins or until a knife inserted in the middle comes out clean. Allow to cool in the pan for 15 mins, then remove from the pan and cool completely on a wire rack.

Whlie the loaf cake is baking, make the icing. Let the butter come to room temperature, until it is soft. Whip the butter in a large bowl until it has doubled in volume, add the icing sugar and cinnamon, and then beat until the icing is thick and creamy. When the cake is cool to the touch, spread the icing on top, then sprinkle with cinnamon in a decorative pattern and drizzle the remaining chopped nuts.

Deviled Eggs (6 Servings)

Per Serving = Calories: 143 – Fat: 12g
– Carbs:2 g – Protein: 6g

Ingredients:

- 6 hard-boiled eggs, halved
- 3 tablespoons mayonnaise
- 1 teaspoon Dijon mustard
- 1 teaspoon vinegar
- 1/8 teaspoon salt
- 1/8 teaspoon pepper
- 12 black olives

Directions:

Cut eggs in half lengthwise. Using a spoon, remove the yolk from the whites, being careful not to ruin the shape of the whites.

Mash the yolks with a fork, stirring in the chopped black olives, the mayonnaise, mustard, vinegar, salt and pepper.

Place the yolks back into the eggs with your spoon or a decorative piping tool. Sprinkle with paprika and serve.

Eggs and Fries (2 Servings)

Per Serving = Calories: 303 – Fat:19 g – Carbs: 25g – Protein: 11g

Ingredients:

- 2 medium baking potatoes, cut into chunky wedges
- 2 T olive oil
- 1 tsp smoked paprika
- 2 tomatoes, halved
- 2 eggs

Directions:

Heat the oven to 375F. Place the potato wedges into a 9 x 13 baking pan. Drizzle the olive oil over the potatoes, stirring to thoroughly coat them. Sprinkle the paprika over the potatoes and stir again. Place in the oven for 25 minutes, partially roasting the potatoes. Pull the potatoes and flip them all with a spatula.

Place the tomatoes, cut side to the upside, in between the potatoes, like a kind of nest. Scooch out the potatoes to allow for space for the two eggs, and crack an egg into each space.

Place back in the oven and cook for 6-8 minutes until the potatoes and eggs are done to your liking.

Florentine Eggs (4 Servings)

Per Serving = Calories: 828 – Fat: 68g – Carbs: 18g – Protein: 37g

Ingredients:

- 8 thin bacon slices
- 1 ounce pat of butter
- 2 bunches spinach, trimmed, washed, dried
- Dash of white vinegar
- 4 fresh eggs, at room temperature
- 4 slices gluten free bread, toasted

Hollandaise sauce

- 1/4 cup white wine vinegar
- 6 black peppercorns
- 2 egg yolks
- 7 ounces unsalted butter, melted
- 2 teaspoons lemon juice

Directions:

Begin with the Hollandaise Sauce:

Combine the vinegar, peppercorns in a small pan over a low flame. Simmer these ingredients for 3-5 minutes, until the liquid is reduced to 2 teaspoons. Remove the pan from the heat and pour the liquid base through a fine colander. Keep the liquid for the hollandaise sauce.

Place the vinegar base and the egg yolks into a double boiler, whisking continually. Add the melted better in a slow stream, while whisking to create an even mix. Whisk until the sauce changes texture from thin to thick and creamy. Season with pepper and salt to taste. Add the lemon juice to the sauce and whisk to combine. Set aside and cover with foil as you prepare the eggs and bacon.

Heat a frying pan over high heat, add the bacon and fry until crisp. Place on a paper towel to drain. Melt the remaining butter in the frying pan until the butter foams. Place the spinach into the pan and saute, 4 minutes or so, until the spinach wilts. Salt and pepper to taste.

To Poach the Eggs:

Heat a large pan over high heat filled with water. Add a dash of vinegar and reduce the heat to a slow simmer. Crack the egg into a cup, gently so as not to bruise the yolk. Use a wooden spoon to stir the water to ripple like a whirlpool. Gently pour the egg into the whirlpool and cook for 2 minutes for a soft centered egg, or longer if you desire.

Using a slotted spoon, transfer the egg onto the plate. Cover with foil to keep warm while cooking the remaining eggs.

Place the toast in a pleasing arrangement onto the serving plates. Spoon first the spinach, then the bacon, and then the eggs onto the toast slices. Pour the hollandaise sauce in a small stream over each plate, then garnish with parsley and a small slice of lemon. Serve immediately with salt and pepper.

Frittata with Spinach and Ham (4 Servings)

Per Serving = Calories: 319 – Fat: 25g – Carbs: 3g – Protein: 20g

Ingredients:

- 1 bunch spinach, trimmed, shredded
- 100g ham, chopped
- 6 eggs
- 1/2 cup pure cream or lactose free milk
- 1/3 cup grated parmesan cheese
- 250g cherry tomatoes, halved

Directions:

Preheat the oven to 375F. Place parchment paper into an 8 x 8 glass pan. Grease the parchment paper and make sure there is a 2 inch overhang on 2 of the sides.

Layer half of the spinach into the pan. Top with half of the ham. Continue to layer the spinach and the ham. There should be four layers total.

Mix the eggs, cheese, and milk or milk substitute into a bowl, combining thoroughly. Add salt and pepper and pour over the top of the spinach and ham. Arrange the tomatoes on top, with the cut sides upturned.

Bake 35 to 40 minutes until golden brown and the eggs are set. Rest 10 minutes before cutting. Serve with gluten free rolls or toast and a small serving of strawberries or raspberries on the side.

Irish Soda Bread (8 Servings)

Per Serving = Calories: 175 – Fat:3 g – Carbs:33 g – Protein: 4g

Ingredients:

- scant 1 cup milk or non-dairy substitute
- 1 tablespoon vinegar or lemon juice
- 1 large egg, lightly beaten
- 1 tablespoon grapeseed oil, light olive oil or canola oil
- 1 1/2 cups white rice flour
- 1/2 cup tapioca starch
- 1 1/2 tablespoons powdered dextrose (or 1 Tbsp. sugar)
- 1 teaspoon baking soda
- 1 teaspoon baking powder
- 1/2 teaspoon salt

Directions:

Preheat oven to 350 degrees F. Grease and flour a 9" cake pan or a 9" x 5" loaf pan.

Place the 1 T vinegar or lemon juice into a glass measuring cup. Pour enough milk into the measuring cup to equal 1 cup total. Stir the two ingredients and let sit for 2 minutes.

Combine the milk mix, the egg and the oil into a medium sized bowl.

In a larger bowl, place the rice flour, tapioca starch, sugar or dextrose, baking powder, baking soda and salt. Mix these together and then add the milk mixture and stir well with a wooden spoon.

Pour into the baking pan and bake for 20-25 minutes until golden brown. Insert a knife into the center to check for doneness.

Cool in the pan for 15 minutes then turn onto a plate and serve warm.

Muesli (4 Servings)

Per Serving = Calories: 367 –
Fat:10g– Carbs: 35g – Protein: 7g

Ingredients:

- 4 cups rice flakes
- 1/2 cup sultanas
- 1/2 cup dried cranberries
- 1/3 cup pumpkin seeds (pepitas)
- 1/3 cup flaked almonds, toasted
- Reduced-fat milk or almond milk, to serve

Combine the flaked almonds, pumpkin seeds, dried cranberries, sultanas, and rice flakes into a large bowl. Gently stir until well combined, then divide into 4 individual portions. Serve this muesli with lactose-tolerant milk.

Oatmeal with Cinnamon Spiced Bananas (6 Servings)

Per Serving = Calories:399 – Fat: 21g – Carbs:45 g – Protein:5 g

Ingredients:

- 2 cups (180g) rolled oats (not instant)
- 1/4 teaspoon ground cinnamon, plus extra to dust
- 125g brown sugar
- 300ml thickened cream or almond milk
- 2 bananas, sliced
- 4 cups plus 2 T water

Directions:

Cook the oats by placing the oats, cinnamon, 4 cups of water and a pinch of salt into a saucepan over medium heat. Bring the oats to a boil and simmer for 3 minutes.

Place the sugar in a separate saucepan with 2 T of water. Stir continuously over low heat until the sugar dissolves. Turn up the heat to medium and cook for 2 or 3 minutes until the sugar has carmelized. Add

2/3 of the cream or almond milk and stir over low heat, until a caramel sauce is made.

Divide the oat porridge into 6 servings. Place the sliced bananas into the caramel sauce and bathe them. Place them on top of the porridge, sprinkle all with cinnamon, and drizzle with the remaining caramel sauce and milk or cream.

PB2 Granola Bars (6 Servings)

Per Serving = Calories: 159 – Fat:5 g – Carbs: 25g – Protein: 5g

Ingredients

- 2/3 cup PB2 powder* (PB2 powder is peanut butter powder, available at any grocery)
- 1/3 cup water
- 3 tablespoons pure maple syrup
- 1 teaspoon vanilla extract
- 1/2 teaspoon ground cinnamon
- 1 cup quinoa flakes or gluten-free quick oats
- 1/3 cup unsweetened flaked coconut
- 2 tablespoons mini chocolate chips (Enjoy Life for dairy-free)

Directions:

Hydrate the PB2 powder with water and mix together until they are of one consistency and creamy. Stir in the vanilla, maple syrup and cinnamon. Add the quinoa flakes (or oats), the coconut, and the chocolate chips. Stir until the mixture sticks together. The mix will be a little dry, but should be sticky and hold together.

Line a small 4 x 8 loaf pan with parchment paper and grease the paper. Press the mixture into the pan with your hands or the back of a spoon. Press firmly.

Place the pan in the refrigerator for at least 3-4 hours. Remove the bars from the pan and cut into 6 slices. Wrap each slice in saran wrap or a sealed sandwich bag and store in the refrigerator.

Velvet Scrambled Eggs (1 Serving)

Per Serving = Calories:254 – Fat: 19g – Carbs:4 g – Protein:18 g

Ingredients:

- 2 large eggs
- 6 T cream
- 2 T butter

Directions:

When making velvety eggs, it's all about the texture.

Whisk the eggs, milk or cream and a dash of salt together and whisk until air pockets form.

Heat a small, non-stick frying pan for a few seconds, then add the butter and let it slowly melt. Don't allow the butter to get hot and smoke or to brown. Pour in the eggs and let them sit without stirring, until the slow count of 20. Stir gently with a wooden spatula, lifting the eggs and folding from the bottom to the top. Do not stir in circles as this will unevenly harden the eggs.

Repeat the folding unti the eggs are almost done to your liking. Take off the flame and allow to sit for a few minutes as eggs continue to cook even when removed from the heat. Serve the eggs while as warm as possible.

Chapter 3: ....Low-FODMAP Lunch/Snack Recipes

Antipasto on a Stick (1 serving)

Per Serving = Calories:263 – Fat: 17g – Carbs:8 g – Protein:22 g

Ingredients

- 1 small jar peperoncini
- 1 small jar pitted Kalamata olives
- fresh mozzarella balls, small, 2 for each skewer
- Thinly sliced ham or Canadian bacon
- Basil leaves or spinach leaves
- grape tomatoes
- skewers about 6 inches long

Directions

Cut the peperoncini in half so that it will fit evenly on the skewer.

Fold the ham into quarters to fit on the skewer.

Layer the ingredients on the skewer, placing 2 mozzarella balls, 2 slices of ham, 1 whole peperoncini, and 2 grape tomatoes on each skewer. Add olives between the ingredients as you desire.

Nutrition Information is based on 5 olives per skewer.

Serve on a platter with spinach leaves scattered around for a beautiful presentation.

Baked Fries (4 Servings)

Per Serving = Calories: 188– Fat: 7g – Carbs: 30g – Protein: 3g

Ingredients:

- 1 tablespoon olive oil
- 3 or 4 potatoes, unpeeled, cut length-wise into 8 wedges
- 2 tablespoons lemon juice
- 1 teaspoon dried oregano
- 1/2 teaspoon kosher salt
- 1/2 teaspoon coarse ground black pepper

Directions:

Preheat the oven to 400 F. Line a large rimmed baking sheet with aluminum foil, shiny side up, and spray with garlic flavored olive oil spray.

Place the potato wedges, olive oil, lemon juice, salt, pepper and oregano into a large bowl and mix well, turning the potatoes several times to ensure they are well coated.

Place the potatoes skin side down onto the cookie sheet.

Bake for 35 to 40 minutes until golden brown.

If you wish for the potatoes to be extra crispy, turn the potatoes after 20 minutes.

BLT Bits (30 Servings)

Per Serving = Calories: 49 – Fat: 5g – Carbs: 0g – Protein: 2g

Ingredients

- 30 cherry tomatoes
- 1 lb. bacon, cooked crisp, drained and crumbled
- 1/2 cup mayonnaise
- 1/3 cup chopped green onion tips
- 2 tablespoons chopped parsley
- 1/4 teaspoon black pepper

Directions:

To prepare the tomatoes, cut each cherry tomato in half and scoop out the pulp and seeds with a rounded ¼ teaspoon measure. Place the tomatoes cut side down to drain on a paper towel.

Combine the remaining ingredients in a bowl and let chill for 30 minutes while the tomatoes are draining.

Take the ¼ rounded teaspoon and scoop the mayonnaise mixture into the tomatoes. To help keep the tomatoes from running away, slice a small tip off the bottom of the tomato. This will make it stay put.

Refrigerate several hours before serving. To make the dish even more attractive, serve with black olives and green stuffed olives.

Chef Salad (4 Servings)

Per Serving = Calories: 689– Fat: 13g
– Carbs:27 g – Protein: 26g

Ingredients

- 8 slices of salami
- 2 hard-boiled eggs, peeled, halved
- 12 cherry tomatoes, halved
- 4 slices of Jarlsberg cheese
- 8 baby potatoes, cooked, halved
- 1 baby romaine
- 1 cup mixed baby salad leaves
- 12 black olives

Crusty gluten free bread rolls, to serve

Dressing

- 2 tablespoons mayonnaise
- 2 tablespoons olive oil
- 1 tablespoon lemon juice
- 1 tablespoon chopped flat-leaf parsley
- 1 teaspoon Dijon mustard

Directions:

To make the dressing, place the ingredients in a bowl, add 2 tsp warm water and whisk until mixed. Add salt and pepper and set to the side.

To make the salad, tear the Romaine into even pieces and toss with the mixed baby salad leaves before placing on the plate. Cut the 8 slices of salami in half and roll each piece to a cone. Place 2 of these on each plate. Cut the 4 slices of cheese into triangles and place 2 on each plate, opposite the salami cones. Place 4 baby potato halves on each plate, and surround with the tomatoes and olives. Drizzle the salad plates with the dressing and place the egg halves in the center of the plate. Serve with crusty rolls.

Chicken Skewers (4 Servings)

Per Serving = Calories: 65 at: Fat: 1g
– Carbs: 3g – Protein: 11g

Ingredients:

- 1 x 225g can pineapple pieces in natural juice, strained, juice reserved
- 2 tablespoons tomato sauce
- 1 tablespoon soy sauce
- 1 large green bell pepper, halved, deseeded, cut into 2cm pieces
- 4 green onions, tips only, chopped
- 12 (about 550g) chicken tenderloins, cut into thirds crossways
- Olive oil spray

Directions:

Make a marinade with the pineapple juice, soy sauce, and tomato sauce in a bowl.

Place the marinade in the refrigerator and add the chicken. Turn to coat the chicken every 15 minutes. Marinate for a total of one hour.

Thread the green bell pepper, pineapple and chicken alternately onto skewers. Spray lightly with olive oil spray.

Preheat a portable grill, barbecue, or large frying pan on medium-high. Place the chicken on the heat and cook, turning occasionally, for 10 minutes or until the chicken is grilled. Serve.

Chowder Base for Soup (6 Servings)

Per Serving = Calories: 369 – Fat: 15g – Carbs: 34g – Protein: 25g

Ingredients:

- 1 medium carrot, finely chopped
- 1 stick celery, finely chopped
- 3 (750g) potatoes, peeled, roughly chopped
- 4 cups (1 litre) Campbell's Real Chicken Stock
- 2 corn cobs
- 500g marinara mix
- 200ml thickened cream or almond milk
- 2 tablespoons chopped fresh chives
- 2 tablespoons chopped fresh parsley

Crusty bread, to serve (Gluten free)

Directions:

To make the soup base, place the carrot, celery, potatoes and chicken stock into a large pot. Cover the pot and bring the contents to a boil. Reduce and simmer the base for 10-15 minutes, until the vegetables are very tender. Place the cooled mixture into a blender and process until smooth. Return to the soup pot.

Cut the kernals from the fresh corn and add it to the soup continue to simmer until the corn is tender and soft, about 10 more minutes.

Reduce the heat to very low and add the marinara mix and the milk. Stir and do not allow to boil. Add your choice of seafood and continue to lightly simmer until the chowder is hot and the seafood is done. Sprinkle with the parsley and chives. Serve while hot. Salt and pepper to taste.

Cod Stuffed Baked Potatoes (4 Servings)

Per Serving = Calories: 375 at: Fat: 12g – Carbs: 41g – Protein: 30g

Ingredients:

- 1 cup (250ml) milk
- 320g smoked cod
- 4 large (about 300g each) Idaho potatoes
- 1 tablespoon olive oil
- 2 hard-boiled eggs, peeled, chopped
- 2 tablespoons chopped chives
- 2 tablespoons grated parmesan

Directions:

Preheat the oven to 400F.

Place milk in a frying pan over medium heat. Add cod, skin-side up, and poach for 7-8 minutes until warm. Remove cod and reserve 1/2 cup milk. Use a fork to flake fish into small pieces, discarding the skin, and place the cod in a bowl and to the side.

Meanwhile, brush potatoes with oil, poke with a fork and place in the microwave. Microwave on high for 12-14 minutes until done (they're ready when a fork is easily inserted). Cool slightly, then cut off the tops for a flat surface. Scoop out the contents of each potato, leaving a thicker wall so the skins hold their shape.

Put the potato shells to the side and place the potato insides in the bowl with the fish. Add egg, chives and reserved poaching milk, then mash lightly and season. Place the filling back into the potato skins and sprinkle the top with parmesan. Bake for 15 minutes or until the cheese is golden.

Crab and Miso Soup (4 Servings)

Per Serving = Calories: 514.50 at:
Fat: 15g – Carbs: 82.60g – Protein:
22.50g

Ingredients:

- 2 x 250g pkts Instant Brown Medium Grain Rice in 90 seconds
- 2 bunches broccolini, stems sliced
- 2 corn cobs
- 1/3 cup white miso paste
- 1/4 cup tahini
- 200g fresh crab meat, cooked
- 1/3 cup chopped chives
- 2 teaspoons black sesame seeds, toasted

Directions:

Cook rice following the package directions.

Meanwhile, place 6 cups of water in a large saucepan. Bring the water to boil over high heat. Add the broccolini and cook for 1 minute. Meanwhile cut corn kernels from the fresh cobs. Add to the pan with rice and cook for 1 minute. Remove from heat. Add miso paste and tahini and stir until well combined. Divide between 4 serving bowls. Add the crab and sprinkle with chives and sesame seeds.

Crockpot Baked Potatoes (4 Servings)

Per Serving = Calories: 172 – Fat: .2g – Carbs: 39g – Protein: 4g

Slow cooker

Ingredients:
- 4 large baking potatoes
- Salt, to season
- Butter, to serve

Directions:

Wash the potatoes thoroughly, then oil the outsides of the potatoes.

Poke the potatoes several places with a fork and roll them in salt.

Wrap each potato with foil and place them seam side up in the slow cooker.

Cook on low for 8 hours, serve with butter, salt and pepper.

Grape and Chicken Salad (4 Servings)

Per Serving = Calories: 272 – Fat:12.8 g – Carbs: 16g – Protein: 23.7g

Ingredients:

- 330g Roasted Chicken
- 1 bunch watercress, washed, trimmed
- 1 fennel bulb, shaved
- 250g red seedless grapes, halved lengthways
- 80ml (1/3 cup) Pomegranate Dressing

Directions:

Slice the roasted chicken into thin pieces. Toss the watercress, fennel, grapes and chicken into a bowl. Place on serving plates and drizzle with the pomegranate dressing.

Greek Style Salad with Crunchy Cucumber (Serves 4)

Per Serving = Calories: 199 at: Fat: 15.9g – Carbs: 7.4g – Protein: 8g

Ingredients:

- 2 cucumbers, partially peeled and sliced longways
- 1 tablespoon olive oil
- 2 teaspoons red wine vinegar
- 2 ounces kalamata olives
- 4 ounces cherry tomatoes, halved
- 7 ounces Feta, halved diagonally
- 1/2 teaspoon dried oregano leaves, to serve
- Pinch dried chili flakes, to serve

Directions:

Peel the cucumber so that you have long stripes on the outside. Slice the cucumber in half longwise and seed it. Slice the remaining cucumber so that you have half moons with an outer stripe.

Whisk the vinegar and oil together until blended.

Place the cucumbers, olives and tomatoes into a bowl and gently toss with the vinegar and oil mixture.

Move the seasoned vegetables onto the serving plates and place the Feta in the middle of the plate. Scoop the vegetables around the cheese and drizzle all with the remaining vinegar and oil. Sprinkle the oregano and chili flakes over the cheese for color.

Hot and Sour Soup (4 Servings)

Per Serving = Calories: 203 at: Fat: 7g – Carbs: 10g – Protein: 22g

Ingredients:

- 1L (4 cups) Campbell's Real Chicken Stock
- 200g pork fillet, slivered
- 5cm piece ginger, peeled and slivered
- 2 tablespoons canned bamboo shoots
- 250g firm tofu, sliced into matchsticks
- 1 tablespoon corn flour
- 2 tablespoons soy sauce
- 2 tablespoons rice vinegar
- 1/2 teaspoon sesame oil
- Chili oil, to serve (optional)

Directions:

Bring the chicken stock to a light boil, then turn the heat to simmer. Add pork, ginger, bamboo shoots and 1/2 teaspoon salt and simmer for 2 minutes, skimming the top of foam. Add tofu and simmer for 2 minutes.

Mix the corn flour with soy sauce and vinegar and add gradually to the soup, stirring continuously to thicken the soup. The soup will be shiny. Stir in 1/2 teaspoon white pepper.

Serve drizzled with sesame oil, and chili oil if desired.

Ketchup (4 Servings)

Per Serving = Calories: 180– Fat: 0g – Carbs: 44g – Protein: 4g

Ingredients:

- 12 oz Tomato Paste
- 1/2 Cup Dark Brown Sugar
- 1/2 teaspoon Dry Ground Mustard
- 1/2 teaspoon Salt
- 1/2 teaspoon Cinnamon
- 1/4 teaspoon Ground Cloves
- 1/4 teaspoon Gluten Free Asafoetida Powder (Garlic & Onion Replacement)
- 1/4 teaspoon Cayenne Pepper
- 2/3 Cup Water
- 4 Tablespoons White Wine Vinegar

Directions:

Mix all ingredients together until the Brown Sugar is completely dissolved.

Store refrigerated in an airtight container. Will keep if refrigerated for 3-4 weeks.

Lemon Romaine Salad with Toasted Pecans (10 Servings)

Per Serving = Calories: 159 – Fat:16 g – Carbs: 2g – Protein: 1.6g

Ingredients:

- 1 pkg romaine lettuce, roughly torn
- 5 sticks celery, sliced diagonally
- 1 cup pecan nuts, toasted, chopped

Lemon dressing

- 1/3 cup olive oil
- 1/4 cup lemon juice
- 1 1/2 teaspoons brown sugar

Directions:

Place all the dressing ingredients and blend until a lovely sunshine color.

Arrange the celery, lettuce and half the nuts in a clear glass bowl. Pour the dressing on top, and stir to mix so that each leaf has a coating of dressing. Sprinkle with the last of the nuts and serve.

Maple Popcorn with Pecans (6 servings)

Per Serving = Calories: 392 – Fat: 28 g – Carbs: 40g – Protein: 4g

Ingredients:

- 6 cups popcorn, air-popped
- 1 cup, chopped, pecans
- 6 tbs, Butter - Salted
- 3/4 cup Brown Sugar Packed
- 2 tbsp Real Maple syrup
- ¼ tsp baking soda
- 1 tsp Vanilla extract
- 1/2 cup Raw Pepitas

Directions:

Preheat oven to 300 degrees. Prepare a cookie sheet by lining it with parchment paper and spraying with butter flavored cooking spray.

Spray a non-stick skillet with butter flavored cooking spray. Place the pumpkin seeds (pepitas) and the pecans in the skillet and toast, stirring constantly until fragrant and roasted. Remove the skillet from the heat.

Pop the popcorn in an air popper. If you don't have an air popper, place 1/3 cup raw popcorn kernels in a paper bag with the top taped lightly with Scotch tape. Place in the microwave. Pop it just until you can no longer hear popping noises, or press the popcorn button. Don't burn the popcorn or it will taste yucky and smell awful.

Spread the popcorn and nuts evenly on the baking sheet. Pick out any widows and orphans (unpopped kernals and half hulls) from the layer on the sheet.

Over medium heat in a large saucepan, add butter, sugar and maple syrup. Stir steadily until the mixture is melted and the syrup is bubbling.

Stop stirring and cook for 5 more minute.

Remove from heat and add in baking soda and vanilla, the mixture will foam up and grow tremendously in size. It will be hot and sticky. Do not get it on your fingers as it will burn and hurt.

Take a wooden spoon and spray with cooking spray, dip into the maple mixture and drizzle maple topping over popcorn. Mix it quite well and spread onto the baking sheets. Make this one layer that is evenly spread. Do not use your fingers for spreading, use two wooden spoons. If you feel you must use fingers, place the ove-glove over your hands and place a layer of waxed paper between your fingers and the popcorn. Place into the oven and bake 15 minutes.

Remove from the oven and allow to cool. This is very hot!

Sprinkle with nutmeg, cinnamon, or cocoa. One cup equals one serving.

Mexican Lime Chicken (4 Servings)

Per Serving = Calories: 204– Fat:10 g – Carbs:1 g – Protein: 26g

Ingredients:

- 1 lb. boneless, skinless chicken breasts, pounded to an even thickness
- 1/4 cup fresh lime juice
- 2 tablespoons olive oil
- 1/2 teaspoon ancho chili powder
- 1/2 teaspoon salt
- 1/4 teaspoon fresh ground black pepper

Directions:

Make a marinade of lime juice, ancho chili powder, salt and pepper. Pour this into a sealable plastic bag or bowl and place the chicken breasts inside, poking them first with a fork so they will absorb more marinade. Refrigerate for two hours, turning the chicken over every 30 minutes to ensure it is coated evenly.

Drain the chicken and grill over medium until the chicken is done.

Oat Encrusted Fish with Salad of Baby Greens (4 Servings)

Per Serving = Calories: 589 – Fat: 20g – Carbs: 45g – Protein: 55g

Ingredients:

- 180g (2 cups) rolled oats
- 1/2 cup chopped fresh parsley
- 2 tablespoons finely grated lemon rind
- 75g (1/2 cup) corn flour
- 2 eggs, lightly whisked
- 4 (about 180g each) firm white fish fillets (such as perch)
- 2 cucumbers
- 1 carrot, peeled, cut into matchsticks
- 65g (1 cup) bean sprouts, trimmed
- Extra light olive oil, to shallow-fry
- 120g baby salad mix
- Tartar sauce, to serve
- Lemon wedges, to serve

Directions:

Clear your work counter and place a plate in the first section, seasoned with the salt and pepper.
Place the egg (whisked in a bowl) in the second section.
In the third, combine the oats, parsley and lemon rind on a large plate.

Take the fish fillets, roll them in the flour, dip into the egg, then place in the oats, pressing the oats to coat the fish firmly. Place on a clean plate and put the fish in the refrigerator to chill for 30 minutes.

Slice the cucumbers into ribbons the size of the carrot matchsticks. Place the cucumber, bean sprouts and carrots into a large bowl.

Heat the oil to fry the fish in a frying pan. Cook half the fish, flip it over, and cook the other half. Turn only one time and cook 4-5 minutes to each side. Place on a paper towel to drain.

Place the fish and baby greens onto a plate, place the cucumber mix atop the greens. Serve with lemon/or tartar sauce.

Pad Thai Noodles (4 Servings)

Per Serving = Calories: 380– Fat: 21g – Carbs: 28g – Protein:16 g

Ingredients:

- 250g rice stick noodles
- 2 tablespoons Rice Oil
- 2 eggs, scrambled a bit
- 1/3 cup pad Thai paste
- 250g firm tofu, chopped into fine pieces
- 100g beansprouts, ends trimmed
- 2 tablespoons peanuts, chopped coarsely
- lime wedges, for garnish

Directions:

Place the rice noodles in a heatproof bowl. Cover with boiling hot water. Stand for 10 minutes until softened. Drain the noodles in a colander. Set the noodles aside.

Heat 1 tablespoon of oil in a large frying pan. Add egg and fry softly, enough that the white is set. Cook for

2 minutes and remove to a plate.
Roughly chop the egg.

Heat the remaining oil in the pan.
Add the Thai paste and tofu. Stir
together in the oil for 1 minute or
until fragrant. Add the rice noodles.
Cook, stirring, for 1 minute or until
the noodles are warmed through.
Remove from heat.

Divide the noodle mixture between
the serving bowls. Place the
beansprouts on top, then the pieces of
egg, then the peanuts. Squirt a spritz
of lime juice into the noodles and
serve with decorative lime pieces.

Parmesan Coated Wings (24 Servings)

Per Serving = Calories: 142 – Fat: 11g – Carbs: 0g – Protein: 11g

Ingredients:

- 24 chicken wings
- olive oil cooking spray
- 1 tablespoon garlic flavored olive oil
- 3 tablespoons butter
- 1/4 teaspoon salt
- 1/4 teaspoon ground black pepper
- 1/2 cup finely shredded Parmesan cheese
- Chopped fresh parsley

Directions:

Preheat oven to 375 degrees F. Line a large baking sheet with aluminum foil, shiny side up, and spritz with olive oil cooking spray. Place the wings on the prepared sheet and season with salt and pepper. Bake for 1 hour, or until golden-brown.

In a small saucepan, heat olive oil. Add butter and melt to combine with the oil. Stir in salt and pepper.

Arrange wings on a serving plate and drizzle with the butter and oil mixture. Sprinkle with Parmesan cheese and chopped parsley and serve.

Pina Colada Bites (4 Servings)

Per Serving = Calories: 460 – Fat: .4g – Carbs: 107g – Protein:1.8 g

Ingredients:

- 1.3kg pineapple
- 1 1/2 cups caster sugar
- 1 cup water
- 1 tablespoons liquid glucose
- 2 teaspoons Coconut extract

Directions:

Cut the pineapple slices into smaller bits.

Combine the sugars and water into a saucepan, stirring until all the sugars are melted. Bring the liquid to a simmer. Add the pineapple and 2 teaspoons coconut extract. Slowly continue to simmer for 40 minutes or until the pineapple is opaque.

Use a slotted spoon to transfer to a rack placed over a baking tray lined with baking paper.

Preheat oven to 225F. Bake for 1 1/4 hours, to dry the pineapple. Allow the pineapple to cool. Store in an airtight container at room temperature or refrigerate if the atmosphere is humid.

Potato Salad (5 Servings)

Per Serving = Calories: 261 – Fat:18 g – Carbs:20 g – Protein: 4g

Ingredients:

- 650g (about 5) red-skinned potatoes, unpeeled, cut into 2.5cm pieces
- 2 tablespoons chopped fresh parsley
- 85g (1/3 cup) mayonnaise
- 2 teaspoons fresh lemon juice
- Salt & freshly ground black pepper

Directions:

Scrub the potatoes well as you will be eating the skins. Place the potatoes in a pot of cold water and cover. Bring the pot to a rolling boil. Reduce the heat to medium and boil, partially covered for 10 minutes or until just tender. Drain and let cool for 30 minutes.

Place the potatoes in a large bowl with the parsley.

Place the mayonnaise and lemon juice in a bowl and mix with salt and pepper to taste.

Add to the potatoes, being gentle so as not to break the potatoes into smaller pieces.

Quinoa and Cucumber Salad (4 Servings)

Per Serving = Calories: 136 – Fat: 3g – Carbs: 21g – Protein: 4.5g

Ingredients:

- 3/4 cup quinoa, rinsed
- 1 1/2 tablespoons lemon juice
- 1 teaspoon extra-virgin olive oil
- 1/3 cup chopped fresh flat-leaf parsley leaves
- 1 small cucumber, peeled, deseeded, diced

Directions:

Place the quinoa and 1 ½ cups cold water in a small pot over high heat. Cover the pot and bring to a boil, reducing the heat to simmer after the bubbles break the surface. Simmer for 12 minutes until the quinoa is done and the water has been absorbed. Drain and rinse the quinoa. Place in a larger bowl.

Mix the lemon juice, oil, parsley, cucumber together in a jar with a lid. Tighten the lid and shake the dressing to combine all the flavors and textures. Pour over the quinoa and toss lightly. Serve.

Quinoa with Almonds and Feta Salad (4 Servings)

Per Serving = Calories: 404 – Fat: 19g – Carbs: 44g – Protein: 17g

Ingredients:

- 1 T olive oil
- 1 tsp ground coriander
- ½ tsp turmeric
- 300g quinoa rinsed
- 50g toasted flaked almonds
- 100g feta cheese, crumbled
- handful parsley roughly chopped
- juice ½ lemon

Heat the oil in a large frying pan. Add the spices, then fry for a minute or two until fragrant. Add the quinoa, then fry for a further minute or two until you can hear gentle popping sounds. Stir in 600ml boiling water, then gently simmer for 10-15 minutess until the water has evaporated and the quinoa grains are done. Allow to cool, then add the almonds, cheese, parsley and lemon juice. Serve warm or cold.

Raspberry-Coconut Bars (16 Servings)

Per Serving = Calories: 169 – Fat: 9g – Carbs: 21g – Protein: 3.7g

8 in square cake pan

Ingredients:

- 2 cups raspberries
- 2 tablespoons lemon juice
- 1/2 cup white chia seeds
- 2 cups rolled oats
- 1 cup shredded coconut
- 1/2 cup macadamia, coarsely chopped
- 1/3 cup pepitas
- 2 tablespoons sesame seeds
- 2/3 cup maple syrup
- 1/3 cup macadamia oil

Directions:

Place raspberries and juice in a small saucepan over medium-high heat. Cook, stirring, occasionally, for 3 minutes or until the raspberries have softened. Remove from heat and stir in the chia seeds. Set the saucepan and fruit aside to cool.

Preheat oven to 275F. Grease and line sides and bottom of an 8 inch square cake pan.

Place the oats, coconut, macadamia nuts, pepitas and sesame seeds in a bowl. Mix the maple syrup and the oil in a saucepan over medium heat for 3 minutes. Pour over the oats mixture and still together.

Spoon half into the square pan, pressing with your well greased hands. Pour the raspberry mix over the oats, then top with the remaining oats. Press well with greased hands.

Bake for 50 minutes. Cool on a wire rack then place in the refrigerator for one hour. Remove from the fridge and cut into 16 squares with a buttered knife.

Rice and Tuna Salad (4 Servings)

Per Serving = Calories: 354 at: Fat: 6g – Carbs: 65g – Protein: 7g

Ingredients:

- 250g microwave brown rice
- 1 cup microwave white rice
- 1/2 cup frozen peas
- 2 tomatoes, diced
- 2 x 185g cans tuna in spring water
- 2 large lemons
- 1 tablespoon olive oil

Directions:

Cook brown rice following package directions. Spread on a tray and set aside to cool. Microwave the white rice following the package directions. Place the frozen peas into the hot rice and stir, then set aside to let the peas thaw as the rice cools.

Place the two rices, the tuna (drained and flaked) and the tomatoes into a large bowl.

Mix the juice of one lemon with the olive oil for a dressing. Stir by shaking in a sealed jar. Pour over the rice/tuna salad and serve with lemon slices.

Salad Niçoise (4 Servings)

Calories 531 Fat 26g Carbs 38g
Protein 35g

Ingredients:

- 12 (about 650g) baby potatoes
- 320g green beans, topped
- 4 eggs
- 60ml (1/4 cup) extra virgin olive oil
- 1 tablespoon red wine vinegar
- 1 teaspoon Dijon mustard
- Pinch of sugar
- 3 (about 250g each) tuna steaks
- 12 cherry tomatoes, halved
- 100g (2/3 cup) kalamata olives
- 1 cup fresh parsley leaves

Directions:

Cook the baby potatoes in a saucepan of boiling water for 10 minutes or until tender. Transfer the potatoes to a chopping board and chop them coarsely. Add the beans to the pan and cook until bright green. Run under cold running water to stop the cooking process. Dip into ice water to crisp the beans so they will be crunchy. Drain well.

Hard boil the eggs, peel and slice.

Whisk together the mustard, oil, vinegar and sugar in a bowl or small blender. Sprinkle liberally with salt and pepper.

Heat a grill to medium-high heat. Add the tuna and cook for 2-3 minutes each side for medium or longer if you prefer. Place to the side and let it rest for at least 5 minutes. Lightly slice the tuna vertically to place onto the salad for eye appeal.

Divide the potato, green beans, egg, tuna, tomato, olives and parsley among the serving bowls. Drizzle the dressing over the tuna and salad. Season with salt and pepper to serve.

Savory Chicken and Rice Muffins (8 Servings)

Per Serving = Calories: 229 – Fat:8 g – Carbs: 18g – Protein: 20g

Ingredients:

- 2/3 cup Basmati Rice
- 250g skinless smoked chicken breast, chopped finely
- 2/3 cup dried tomatoes, coarsely chopped
- 1 1/3 cups grated fresh mozzarella cheese
- 3 green onions, thinly sliced, the green tops only
- 1/4 cup basil leaves, chopped finely
- 3 eggs, lightly beaten

Directions:

Preheat oven to 400F. Grease Texas sized muffin tin. Line the muffin tin with liners.

Cook the basmati rice as the package suggests. Rinse the rice and let cool.

Place all ingredients into a bowl, with the exception of 1/3 cups of the mozzarella cheese.

Spoon the mixture of chicken and rice into the prepared muffin pan. Sprinkle with remaining cheese. Bake for 15 to 20 minutes or until the muffins are firm and light golden in color. Stand in pan for 5 minutes. Dump the muffins onto a plate and allow to cool. Store in an airtight container. Refrigerate until ready to serve. Enjoy for breakfast or as a light tea snack.

Smoked Salmon Appetizers (20 Servings)

Per Serving = Calories: 12 – Fat: 4g – Carbs: 3g – Protein: 2g

Ingredients:

- 2 large baking potatoes
- 2 tbsp olive oil
- grated zest and juice ½ lemon
- 1 egg yolk
- 140g smoked salmon, plus extra for gnoshing
- 1 tbsp chopped parsley
- 2 tbsp gluten-free flour mixed with 1 tsp coarsely ground pepper
- oil, for frying
- grape tomatoes, for garnish

Directions:

Microwave potatoes on high for 10-12 mins until fork tender. Let cool for 5 mins, scoop out the insides into a bowl, smash with a fork and flavor with olive oil, a sprinkle of lemon juice and the zest, and then add the egg, salmon and parsley. Shape into small cakes with a large tablespoon and place in the fridge to chill.

Sprinkle each cake with the peppered flour, then fry over a low heat in a little oil for 2-3 mins on each side. Drain on a paper towel. Serve warm with a halved grape tomato and parsley for color.

Spinach and Butternut Squash Salad (6 Servings)

Per Serving = Calories: 211 – Fat: 17g – Carbs: 9.5g – Protein: 4.5g

Ingredients:

- 600g butternut squash, peeled and sliced into bites
- 2 teaspoons olive oil
- 2 teaspoons honey
- 2 teaspoons sesame seeds
- 1 tablespoon fresh lemon juice
- 4 tsp brown sugar
- 2 tablespoons extra virgin olive oil
- 2 teaspoons wholegrain mustard
- 1 x 150g pkt baby spinach leaves
- 1 x 75g pkt toasted pine nuts

Directions:

Preheat oven to 425F. Line a baking tray with parchment paper. Place the pieces of squash in a bowl, drizzle with the oil and 3 tsp of the brown sugar. Sprinkle with salt and pepper.

Place the squash onto the baking tray and into the oven. Bake for 25 minutes or until golden brown, turning once during cooking. Remove from the oven and sprinkle evenly with the sesame seeds. Return to the oven and bake for 5 minutes or until the seeds are lightly toasted. Remove from the oven and set aside for 30 minutes to cool.

Combine the lemon juice, olive oil, mustard and extra honey in a small blender and whir until well combined. Season with salt and pepper.

Place all the ingredients into a serving bowl. Drizzle with the dressing and gently toss until just combined. Serve immediately.

Spring Soup (4 servings for an appetizer, 2 for dinner)

Per Serving = Calories:124 – Fat: 7 g – Carbs:10 g – Protein:6 g

Ingredients

1 tablespoon olive oil

4 spring onions, green tops only, diced

2 large handfuls of spinach, diced into small ribbons

2 tablespoons green peas, fresh or frozen

1 cup fresh green beans, sliced into 1 inch pieces

4 c Vegetable stock

1/3 cup gluten free small pasta

½ cup parmesan, grated

Directions

Cook the pasta in 2 cups boiling water, with the olive oil spread into the water.

Remove the pasta from the stove when al dente. Drain the pasta.

Combine 4 cups vegetable stock, and the rest of the ingredients, excluding the cheese.

Simmer for 10 minutes on the stove until the green beans are crisp, but not raw.

Serve in warm bowls and top with the parmesan cheese.

Tuesday Tacos (4 Servings)

Per Serving = Calories: 390 – Fat:20 g – Carbs: 11g – Protein: 41g

Ingredients:

- 1 jalapeno chilies (diced) optional
- 1 handful chives (diced)
- 2 red pepper (green and, diced)
- 2 lbs ground chicken (or turkey)
- 1 can diced tomatoes (with or without chilies)
- 2 tbsps cumin
- 2 tbsps paprika
- 1 tbsp cayenne pepper
- 1 tbsp oregano

Directions:

Start with placing the chives, bell pepper pieces and the ground chicken, with a tablespoon of olive into a skillet and beginning to fry.

Fry the meat and the peppers until the meat is no longer pink, the meat is crumbled, and the peppers are soft.

Sprinkle spices into your meat and mix, tasting occassionally for flavor. When the meat has the desired flavor,

add the can of diced tomatoes and
serve.

Turkey Burgers with Spinach and Feta (4 Servings)

Per Serving = Calories: 360– Fat:24 g – Carbs: 9g – Protein: 28g

Ingredients:

- 1 lb ground turkey
- 1 egg beaten
- 1 cup crumbled feta cheese
- 3 cups frozen spinach, defrosted
- Spices of your choice: paprika, oregano, cayenne pepper, salt, pepper
- Olive oil or your choice of cooking oil

Directions:

Place all the ingredients into one bowl and mix together. Scoop one pattie together and press until firm. Place gently into the cooking oil in a skillet on medium. Place each pattie into the pan in this manner. Let the patties cook for 7 minutes on one side, then gently turn so the patties will stay firm and shaped. Flip the patties and

cook for another 6 or 7 minutes.
Serve

Chapter 4: .... Low-FODMAP Dinner Recipes

Bacon Wrapped Chicken Thighs with Spicy Rice (4 Servings)

Per Serving = Calories: 803 at: Fat 42g – Carbs: 43g – Protein: 63g

Ingredients:

- 8 strips bacon
- 8 skinless chicken thigh fillets
- 2 tablespoons olive oil
- 1 cup White Long Grain Rice
- 1 teaspoon ground turmeric
- 1 small lemon, rind grated, juiced
- 2 cups Campbell's Real Stock Chicken
- 1/4 cup coriander leaves

Directions:

Preheat oven to 350F. Lay bacon flat on a board and cut a piece off each end. Wrap the remaining length of bacon around each chicken thigh, securing with a toothpick.

Place the chicken in a frying pan with the olive oil over medium heat. Fry for two minutes on each side. The bacon will be golden colored.

Add the rice and bacon ends to the frying pan, reducing the heat to low. Cook for 1 minute while the bacon browns and seasons the rice. Add the turmeric, lemon rind, chicken stock, salt and pepper. Cook for 1 additional minute, stirring until well mixed.

Place this rice mix into a casserole dish that is oven-proof and has a cover. Place chicken on top, pressing gently into the rice. Cover with a tight lid or foil.

Bake for 50 minutes.

Remove from the oven and drizzle with the coriander and lemon juice. Remove the toothpicks and serve with the rice.

Baked Tilapia with Roasted Vegetable Assortment (2 Servings)

Per Serving = Calories: 387 – Fat:17 g – Carbs: 28g – Protein: 28g

Ingredients:

- 300g red-skinned potatoes, thinly sliced into rounds
- 1 red pepper, cut into strips
- 2 tbsp extra virgin olive oil
- 1 rosemary sprig, leaves removed and very finely chopped
- 2 tilapia fillets
- 25g pitted black olives, halved
- ½ lemon sliced thinly into rounds
- handful basil leaves

Directions:

Heat oven to 350F. Arrange the potato and pepper slices on a large baking pan covered with non-stick foil. Drizzle over 1 tbsp oil and sprinkle with the rosemary and a pinch of salt and pepper. Toss everything together well and roast for

25 mins, turning the vegetables when halfway through, baking until the potatoes are golden and crisp at the edges.

Arrange the fish fillets on top and scatter the olives over the fish. Place a couple of lemon slices on top of the fish and drizzle with the remaining oil. Bake for a further 7-8 mins until the fish is cooked well. Serve with basil leaves arranged throughout.

Beef Tips in Red Wine Sauce (4 Servings)

Per Serving = Calories: 300 – Fat: 19g – Carbs: 9g – Protein: 23g

Ingredients:

- 1 lb. beef stew meat, cubed
- 2 tablespoons gluten-free flour
- 1/2 teaspoon salt
- 1/4 teaspoon black pepper
- 1 tablespoon olive oil
- 1 clove garlic, smashed,
- 1 tablespoon unsalted butter
- 1/4 cup dry red wine
- 1 cup Low-FODMAP Beef Broth (plus more if necessary)

Directions:

In a large sealable plastic bag, combine the meat, flour, salt and pepper. Shake to coat the meat.

Heat oil in a large skillet over medium-high heat. Add the meat and brown on all sides, turning to ensure even cooking and a crusty surface.

Reduce heat to medium-low and add the butter. Place the meat on a plate and keep warm.

Deglaze the pan with the wine, scraping around to incorporate the beef crust. Let simmer to reduce the wine slightly. Add in the beef and broth. Cover and simmer on low for 1 1/2 to 2 hours, or until meat is tender. Add more beef broth if necessary.

California Sushi Rolls (12 Servings)

Per Serving = Calories: 233   at: Fat 8g – Carbs: 33g – Protein:5g

sushi mat for rolling.

Ingredients:

- 1 cup sushi rice
- 1/4 cup sushi seasoning
- 2 tablespoons mayonnaise
- 2 teaspoons wasabi paste
- 3 nori sheets
- 1 avocado, peeled, cut into strips
- 1 medium red bell pepper, cut into strips
- 170g can crab meat, drained

Directions:

Rinse and drain rice 3 times or until water runs clear. Place rice in a colander. Let drain for 10 minutes.

Place rice and 1 cup cold water in a saucepan over medium heat. Cover and bring to a hard boil. Reduce the heat to low. Simmer, covered, for 12 minutes or until rice is done. Remove from heat. Let stand, covered, for 10 minutes. Transfer to a large ceramic dish. Stir rice with a plastic spatula to break up the lumps. Gradually add seasoning while lifting and turning rice until rice is almost cold.

Combine mayonnaise and wasabi in a bowl.

Place 1 nori sheet, shiny-side down, on sushi mat. Using damp fingers, spread 1/2 cup rice over nori, leaving a small strip at 1 short end. Spread 3 teaspoons mayonnaise mixture across centre of rice. Arrange 1/3 avocado, red pepper and crab over rice. Using sushi mat, roll up firmly to form a roll. Cut roll into 4 slices. Repeat with remaining ingredients to make 12 pieces.

Cheesy Spinach and Quinoa (4 Servings)

Per Serving = Calories: 577 – Fat: 32g – Carbs: 33g – Protein: 40g

Ingredients:

- 1 cup, Quinoa
- 1.50 cup, Chicken, canned, without broth
- 1 tablespoon, Garlic flavored Olive Oil
- 2.67 oz, Baby Spinach
- 1/2 cup, Lactose Free Milk
- 1 large, Egg, whole, cooked, fried
- 1/4 tsp Butter
- 1/4 tsp Teriyaki Pepper Steak seasoning
- 1 1/2 cup shredded cheddar cheese

Directions:

Preheat the oven to 350 degrees F.

Bring the chicken broth to a boil , add the quinoa and cover. Simmer for 15 to 20 minutes, until quinoa is tender and liquid is absorbed.

Meanwhile, in a large skillet, heat olive oil over medium heat. Add the spinach leaves and saute just until spinach is wilted, about 1 to 2 minutes.

Stir the sauteed spinach into the cooked quinoa. Stir together the milk, egg, salt and pepper in a small bowl. Add the milk and egg mixture and 1 cup of the shredded cheese to the quinoa and stir well.

Pour into a lightly greased 1.5 quart casserole dish and bake, uncovered, for 30 minutes. Sprinkle with the remaining 1/2 cup cheese and bake until melted, about 5 more minutes. Serve.

Chicken and Tomatoes in Cream Sauce (4 Servings)

Per Serving = Calories: 262 – Fat: 12g – Carbs: 2g – Protein: 37g

Ingredients:

- 1 tbsp olive oil
- 4 boneless skinless chicken breast
- 200g pack cherry tomatoes
- 3 tbsp pesto
- 3 tbsp almond milk
- fresh basil

Directions:

Heat the oil in a non-stick frying pan. Add the chicken and fry, not turning it until it takes on a bit of color. Flip the chicken and cook on the other side. Continue cooking for 12-15 mins until the chicken is cooked through. Season all over with a little salt and pepper.

Halve the tomatoes and toss them into the pan, stirring them until they start to soften. Reduce the heat and stir in the pesto and milk until it makes a sauce. Scatter with a few basil leaves if you have them, then serve with rice and salad.

Chinese Eggplant (3 Servings)

Per Serving = Calories: 220– Fat: 12g – Carbs: 27g – Protein: 4g

Ingredients:

- 1 pound (or 2) Chinese (long) eggplant, sliced into quarters
- 1/4 teaspoon salt
- 1 teaspoon cornstarch, plus ¼ cup more to coat eggplant
- 1 tablespoon safflower oil
- 1 ½ tablespoons gluten-free soy sauce (tamari)
- 1 tablespoon gluten-free fish sauce
- 1/16 teaspoon wheat-free asafetida powder
- 2 teaspoons turbinado sugar
- 1 1/2 tablespoons sesame oil
- 1 teaspoon minced (fresh or dry) ginger
- 3 scallions, chopped, green tips only

Directions:

Spread sliced eggplant on a paper towel and sprinkle salt on both sides of eggplant slices. Allow to rest for 1 hour to draw the water out of the eggplant. Pat eggplant dry but do not rinse.

Combine soy sauce, fish sauce, asafetida powder, sugar and 1 teaspoon cornstarch in a bowl and mix well.

Sprinkle ¼ cup cornstarch over the eggplant until the eggplant is evenly coated. Add more cornstarch if needed to coat both sides evenly, making sure each piece of the eggplant is coated.

Heat the oil in a non-stick skillet. Add in ginger and 2 chopped scallions and the sauce. Place eggplant across the surface of the skillet and do not overlap pieces. Grill eggplant pieces until charred and soft, about 8 -10 minutes per side. Transfer to a plate.

Classic Roast Beef with Vegetables (6 Servings)

Per Serving = Calories: 926 at: Fat 51g – Carbs: 34g – Protein: 80g

Ingredients:

- 2 tablespoons butter, at room temperature
- 6 teaspoons olive oil
- 1 2kg rib eye roast
- Salt & freshly ground black pepper
- 1.5kg (about 10) white potatoes, peeled, halved lengthways, patted dry with paper towel
- 2 bunches baby carrots, trimmed to 1cm, washed, scrubbed, patted dry with paper towel
- 1 tablespoon gluten-free flour
- 375ml (1 1/2 cups) Campbell's Real Stock Beef
- Steamed spinach or green beans, to serve

Directions:

Preheat oven to 425F. Heat 2 teaspoons of the butter and 2 teaspoons oil in a large shallow skillet over high heat. Cook the roast, turning occasionally, for 5 minutes or until well browned.

Remove skillet from heat and season beef all over with salt and pepper.

Place the potatoes, 3 teaspoons of the remaining butter and 1 teaspoon of the remaining oil in a bowl. Put disposable gloves on your hands (you will thank me later!) and use your hands to rub the butter and oil evenly over the potatoes. Season the potatoes with salt and pepper. Arrange the potatoes in a single layer around the beef.

Cook beef and potatoes in the preheated oven for 30 minutes, basting beef with the pan juices once during cooking to keep the beef moist.

Place remaining oil and butter in another roasting pan or roasting skillet. Place this pan in the oven for 5 minutes or until butter melts. Add carrots and toss the carrots in the butter to coat well. Turn the potatoes and baste the beef in their roaster. Now add the carrots to the oven and cook, shaking the carrot pan occasionally, for 25 minutes or until the beef is medium or cooked to your liking.

Transfer beef to a large plate and cover loosely with foil. Set aside for 15 minutes to rest. While beef is resting, transfer the potatoes to a tray lined with aluminum foil. Increase oven temperature to 475F. Return potatoes to oven and continue to cook while beef is resting. To make gravy, strain pan juices from the roasting pan into a heatproof container. Return 2 tablespoons of pan juices to a saucepan and heat over high heat. Mix the flour with hot water until it makes a smooth paste. Add this paste to the broth/juices and stir. Cook until thickens, constantly stirring.

Gradually add the stock and cook, scraping the pan with a flat-bottomed wooden spoon to dislodge any bits cooked onto the base of the pan.

Slice the beef across the grain and serve with the gravy, roast potatoes, roast carrots and steamed spinach or beans.

 Add crusty rolls and a tasty dessert for a special family meal.

Fried Rice (4 Servings)

Per Serving = Calories: 356 at: 13.4g
– Carbs: 7.4g – Protein:8g

Ingredients:

- 1 cup White Long Grain Rice
- 2 eggs
- 2 teaspoons vegetable oil
- 2 bacon slices, chopped
- 1 carrot, peeled and grated
- 1 tablespoon soy sauce, plus extra to serve

Directions:

Wash the rice three times and drain, watching to see if the water runs clear. Add the one cup of rice to two cups of water in a saucepan with a lid. Bring to a boil, place a lid on the rice, and reduce the heat to simmer. Cook for 15 minutes. Allow the rice to cool.

Using a whisk, lightly beat eggs in a small bowl. Heat oil in a non-stick wok or frying pan over medium heat. Add eggs. Swirl the eggs over the base to form an omelette. Cook 2 minutes.

Turn over. Cook 2 minutes more until set. Transfer eggs to a chopping board. Let it cool slightly. Cut egg into short strips.

Add the bacon to wok. Cook 4 minutes until light golden. Add the carrot. Stir fry 1 minute. Add the rice. Cook, stirring, 3-4 minutes. Add the chopped egg and soy sauce. Stir until heated through. Serve immediately, with extra soy sauce so each guest can season to taste.

Gingery Egg Drop Soup (4 Servings)

Per Serving = Calories: 112 – Fat: 7g – Carbs: 5g – Protein: 7g

Ingredients:

- 4 cups (1 quart or 946 ml) chicken stock
- 1 1/2 (375 ml) cups water
- 2 tablespoons coconut aminos (or gluten free soy sauce)
- 1 tablespoon minced ginger
- 1/4 teaspoon red chili flakes
- 1 teaspoon fish sauce*
- 2 eggs whisked
- 1/2 cup (1 bunch) spring onions chopped, green parts only
- 2 large zucchini's sliced and diced
- salt & pepper to taste

Directions:

Place the stock, water, coconut aminos, ginger, red chili flakes, and fish sauce in a large sauce pan and heat on a medium high heat.

While the broth is heating, whisk the eggs. Once the broth begins to boil, drizzle the eggs into the soup and stir with a fork or a whisk to create ribbons from the eggs and prevent clumping.

Reduce the heat and then add the spring onions and zucchini and let the soup cook an extra minute or so to soften the zucchini. Season with salt and pepper. Sprinkle with the spring onions and serve.

Greek Chicken (6 Servings)

Calories 644 Fat 33g Carbs 23g
Protein 60g

Ingredients:

- 1 tablespoon olive oil
- 6 small (about 600g) chicken drumsticks
- 6 (about 1.5kg) chicken thigh cutlets
- 1kg new potatoes, halved
- 2 ripe tomatoes, finely chopped
- 95g (1/2 cup) kalamata olives
- 2 sprigs fresh rosemary, leaves picked
- 125ml (1/2 cup) dry white wine
- salt
- black pepper

Directions:

Preheat oven to 400F. Heat the oil in (12-cup capacity) ovenproof baking dish over medium heat. Add the chicken drumsticks and cook, turning occasionally, for 5 minutes or until browned all over. Place to the side but keep warm. Cook the chicken thigh cutlets in the same manner. Transfer them to a plate and cover.

Add the potato to the same dish and cook, turning occasionally, for 5 minutes or until golden. Remove from heat. Add the chicken to the potato in the dish and top with tomatoes and olives. Sprinkle with rosemary. Pour the wine over the chicken and potatoes. Season with salt and pepper.

Bake in oven for 45 minutes or until the chicken is cooked through and the potatoes are tender. Serve immediately.

Lemon-Herb Topped Tilapia with Baby Greens and Basmati Rice (4 Servings)

Per Serving = Calories: 339– Fat: 8g – Carbs: 18g – Protein:45 g

Ingredients:

- 4 slices gluten-free bread, crusts removed
- 2 tablespoons chopped basil leaves
- 2 teaspoons chopped thyme leaves
- 2 tablespoons grated parmesan
- Grated zest of 1/2 lemon
- 1 egg white, lightly beaten
- 4 x 175g tilapia fillets
- 1 tablespoon olive oil
- 2 cups mixed salad leaves
- Basmati rice

Directions:

Preheat the oven to 400F. Line a baking tray with foil, then lightly grease.

Toast the bread until crunchy in the oven. Allow the bread to cool and then grate into crumbs. Add herbs, parmesan, lemon zest and egg white, season with salt and pepper, then mix until just combined.

Brush the top of each fish fillet with a little oil and press some crumb mixture onto each fillet. Transfer to the baking tray. Bake for 10-12 minutes until the fish is cooked through and the topping is golden. Remove from the oven, cover loosely with foil and rest for 5 minutes.

Meanwhile, cook the Basmati rice in a cooking pot according to the package directions for 4 servings. Place onto plates along side the fish and the salad.

Lemon Pepper Chicken and Rice (4 Servings)

Per Serving = Calories: 487 – Fat: 18g – Carbs:17g – Protein: 59g

Ingredients:

- 4 boneless, skinless chicken breasts, sliced thin
- 1 tablespoon Lemon Pepper Seasoning,
- 1/4 cup butter
- 14 oz. unsalted chicken broth
- 1 cup basmati rice
- 1/2 teaspoon salt

Directions:

Preheat oven to 350 degrees F. Select a baking pan with a tight oven-proof lid.

Season chicken breasts with lemon pepper seasoning, sprinkling both sides liberally.

Pour the butter that has been melted into a 13 x 9-inch baking pan. Add the seasoned chicken. Cover with foil, making sure the seal is tight.

Bake for 15 minutes, take the chicken out of the oven, turn it over so the chicken browns nicely, now cook for another 15 minutes.

Remove the chicken from the pan, place to the side. Mix together the remaining ingredients and bake, tightly covered, for 30 minutes.

Take the rice mixture out of the over, place the chicken breasts on top, cover and bake 15 more minutes. Taste the rice to assure it is done. Serve with parsley as a garnish.

New Potato Salad with Green Beans and Anchovies (1 Serving)

Per Serving = Calories: 174 – Fat:5 g – Carbs:20 g – Protein: 9g

Ingredients:

- 4 small eggs
- 100g green beans
- 100g new potatoes
- 1 anchovy finely chopped
- 1 tbsp chopped parsley
- 1 tbsp chopped chives
- juice ½ lemon

Directions:

Bring a medium pan of water to a simmer. Lower the eggs into the water and cook for 2 mins. Lift out the eggs and put into a bowl of cold water and ice cubes. This will make the shells peel easily and will also stop the eggs from cooking. Add the beans to the pan, simmer for 4 mins until tender, then remove from the pan with a slotted spoon and plunge into the bowl of cold water to crisp.

Put the potatoes in the pan and boil for 10-15 mins until tender. Drain the potatoes in a colander and leave them to cool. While the potatoes are cooling, peel the eggs and cut them in half. Toss the potatoes and beans with the chopped anchovy, herbs and lemon juice. Place the eggs on top of the beans and potatoes to serve.

Roasted Leg of Lamb (6 Servings)

Calories 814 Fat 40g Carbs 25g Protein 87g

Ingredients:

- 2kg leg of lamb
- 1 lemon, halved
- 2 1/2 tablespoons olive oil
- 6 brushed white potatoes, peeled, cut into thirds
- 1 tablespoon dried oregano
- 1 bunch baby carrots, trimmed
- salt

Directions:

Preheat oven to 425F. Place the leg of lamb in a large baking dish. Use a sharp knife to make 10 x 3-inch cuts into lamb.

Juice 1 lemon half into a bowl with the 1 tablespoon oil, salt and pepper. Cut remaining lemon into 10 small pieces and push lemon pieces into the cuts. Brush lamb with oil mixture and roast for 15 minutes.

In remaining oil, toss potatoes, oregano, salt and pepper. Arrange potatoes around lamb. Return to oven and roast for 40 minutes.

Add carrots to roasting pan with lamb and potatoes. Roast a further 20 minutes. Remove lamb from oven. Increase oven temperature to 450F. Cook potatoes and carrots a further 15 minutes or until crisp. Cover lamb loosely with foil and rest for 15 minutes.

Carve lamb, reserving 400g for the Shepherd's Pie (see related recipe). Serve with potatoes and carrots.

Shepherd's Pie (4 Servings)

Calories 551 Fat 25g Carbs 40g
Protein 40g

Ingredients:

- 800g potatoes, quartered
- 20g butter
- 1/2 cup hot milk
- 1 1/2 tablespoons olive oil
- 1 carrot, finely chopped
- 1 celery stick, finely chopped
- 1 zucchini, finely chopped
- 400g roast lamb (from Greek-style Roast Lamb - see related recipe), minced
- 1/2 cup tomato sauce
- 2 tablespoons Worcestershire sauce
- 3/4 cup Campbell's Real Beef Stock
- 1/3 cup grated cheddar cheese

Directions:

Cook potatoes until tender. Drain.
Add butter and mash until smooth.
Add milk and beat to combine.

Heat oil in a large, heavy frying pan over medium heat. Cook carrot, celery, zucchini, onion and garlic for 8 to 10 minutes or until vegetables soften.

Add lamb mince, sauces and beef stock. Cook, stirring, until mixture comes to the boil. Simmer for 3 minutes. Set aside to cool.

Preheat oven to 400F. Spoon mixture into 4 x 1-cup ramekins or 1 x 4-cup ovenproof dish. Top with mashed potato. Rake the surface with a fork to create a pattern. Sprinkle with cheese. Bake for 15 to 20 minutes or until golden.

Shrimp Scampi (4 Servings)

Per Serving = Calories: 228 – Fat:16 g
– Carbs: 2g – Protein: 16g

Ingredients:

- 1 tablespoon olive oil*
- 1/4 cup dry white wine
- 1 tablespoon chopped fresh parsley
- 1 1/2 teaspoons lemon juice
- 1 teaspoon Dijon mustard
- 1/4 teaspoon salt
- 1/4 teaspoon black pepper
- 1pound raw shrimp, peeled and deveined, tails left on if desired

Directions:

Preheat oven to 450 degrees F.

Heat oil over medium heat. Add the butter and stir to melt. Add the remaining ingredients except the shrimp. Stir until thoroughly mixed.

Place shrimp in an 8"x 8" baking dish. Pour butter mixture over top.

Bake 12 to 15 minutes or until shrimp are pink and opaque.

Chapter 5: ....Low-FODMAP Dessert Recipes

Almond Cake with Fruit Compote (10 Servings)

Calories 460 Fat 34g Carbs 30g Protein 8g

Ingredients:

- 250g butter, softened
- 2/3 cup caster sugar
- 4 eggs
- 2 cups almond meal (ground almonds)
- 1/4 cup rice flour
- Double cream, to serve

Blueberry and vanilla bean syrup

- 1 vanilla bean, split
- 1/2 cup caster sugar
- 1 cup blueberries

Directions:

Preheat oven to 300F. Grease a springform cake pan. Line base and sides with parchment paper.

Using an electric mixer, beat butter and sugar until light and fluffy. Add eggs, 1 at a time, beating after each addition. Stir in almond meal and flour. Spread mixture into prepared pan. Bake for 1 hour 15 minutes or until a toothpick inserted into the center comes out clean. Stand in pan for 10 minutes, then turn onto a rack to cool.

Meanwhile, to make syrup: Using a sharp knife, scrape seeds from bean. Place seeds, bean, sugar and 1/2 cup cold water in a saucepan over medium heat. Cook, stirring, for 3 minutes or until sugar dissolves (don't boil). Bring to the boil. Reduce heat to low. Simmer for 7 minutes or until slightly thickened. Add blueberries and simmer for 2 to 3 minutes. Very gently stir so as not to break the blueberries. Remove from heat and discard bean.

Place cake on a plate. Spoon blueberry compote onto the cake..

Blueberry Coconut Ice Cream (1 Liter)

Per Serving = Calories: 260– Fat: 16.4g – Carbs: 28.5g – Protein: 3.5g

Ingredients:

- 2 x 270ml cans coconut milk
- 125g fresh blueberries
- 2 teaspoons liquid glucose
- 40g (1/4 cup) coconut sugar
- 1 teaspoon vanilla extract
- 4 egg whites
- 130g (1/3 cup) liquid glucose

Directions:

Two days before you plan to make the ice cream:

Place coconut milk in the fridge for 4 hours or overnight to firm.

One day before you plan to SERVE the ice cream:

Place the blueberries, glucose, 2 tsp of the coconut sugar and half the vanilla in a saucepan over medium-low heat. Cook, stirring occasionally, for 6 minutes or until sugar dissolves and blueberries release their juices. Place in a bowl to cool for 30 minutes. Place in the fridge to cool completely.

Carefully open cans of coconut milk. Scoop the solidified coconut milk from the surface and place in a glass bowl to measure 220ml (reserve remaining liquid for another use). Use a whisk to whisk the solidified coconut milk until thickened slightly.

Use electric beaters with whisk attachment to whisk room temperature egg whites in a clean, dry bowl until firm peaks form. Place the extra glucose and remaining sugar and vanilla in a small saucepan over low heat. Cook, stirring constantly, for 2 minutes or until sugar is almost all dissolved. Bring to a simmer. Simmer, without stirring, until mixture reaches 118C on a sugar thermometer. With the motor running slowly on the mixer, add hot syrup to the egg white, whisking constantly until all combined. Continue whisking for a further 4 minutes or until very thick and bowl is warm to touch. Stand at room temperature for 2 minutes to cool slightly. Use a whisk to fold in whipped coconut milk until smooth.

Pour half the coconut mixture into a 1.4L loaf pan. Spoon two-thirds of the blueberry syrup randomly over top of coconut mixture. Use a butter knife to create a swirled effect. Pour the remaining coconut mixture over the blueberries. Spoon over the remaining blueberry mixture onto the coconut mixture. Use a butter knife to create a swirled effect. Place in the freezer for 8 hours or until firm.

The day you plan to SERVE the ice cream:

Stand the ice-cream at room temperature for 10 minutes before serving.

Brie with Raspberry Compote (4 Servings)

Calories 109 Fat 9g Carbs 6.9g Protein 7.2g

Ingredients:

- 12 fresh raspberries
- 125g round mini brie wheel
- Fresh lemon thyme sprig, to serve
- Sourdough bread, toasted, to serve

Directions:

Preheat oven to 350F. Lightly grease a (1 cup) ramekin. Arrange the berries in the base of the ramekin to cover. Unwrap the brie and place the brie on top.

Bake for 10 minutes or until the brie is warmed through. Turn out onto a serving plate and top with fresh lemon thyme. Serve warm with sourdough toast.

Choco-Chia Peanut Butter Pudding (2 Servings)

Per Serving = Calories: 360 – Fat: 19g – Carbs: 40g – Protein: 14g

Ingredients

- 1 cup dairy free milk of your choice
- ¼ cup chia seeds
- 3 tablespoons cocoa powder
- 1 teaspoon vanilla extract
- 2 tablespoons peanut butter
- 1-2 tablespoons honey

Directions:

Place all of the ingredients into a blender and blend until smooth. Place in a container in the refrigerator overnight and enjoy in the morning for breakfast, or after dinner for dessert.

Chocolate Cobbler 6 Servings

Calories 518 Fat 9g Carbs 103g
Protein 4g

Ingredients:

- 1 cup gluten-free self-rising flour
- 3/4 cup caster sugar
- 1/2 cup cocoa powder, sifted
- 1/2 cup milk
- 1 teaspoon vanilla extract
- 30g butter, melted
- 3/4 cup firmly packed brown sugar
- 1 3/4 cups boiling water
- Double-thick cream and gluten-free icing sugar, to serve

Directions:

Preheat oven to 350F. Lightly grease an 8 cup-capacity oven-proof dish.

Combine flour, caster sugar and 2 tablespoons cocoa in a bowl. Add milk, vanilla and butter. Stir or mix with electric mixer to combine. Pour mixture into prepared pan. Smooth the top so that it seems level.

Combine brown sugar and remaining cocoa in a small bowl. Sift sugar mixture over flour mixture. Pour boiling water over the back of a large metal spoon to cover sugar mixture. Bake for 45 minutes or until a skewer inserted around the edge of cobbler comes out clean. Dust with icing sugar. Serve with cream, if tolerated.

Crunchy Chocolate and Raspberry Parfait (4 Servings)

Per Serving = Calories: 297 – Fat: 11g – Carbs: 43g – Protein: 5g

Ingredients:

- 250g (pint) raspberry
- 2 tbsp Cointreau (or Grand Marnier)
- zest and juice from 1 small orange
- 100g pack dairy, gluten and wheat-free, 'Free From' chocolate
- 3 tbsp soya milk
- 50g caster sugar
- 6 tbsp gluten, wheat and nut-free muesli

Directions:

Divide the raspberries between 4 glasses. Sprinkle ½ tbsp of Cointreau and a little orange zest and juice over each, then set aside.

Melt the chocolate and stir into the soya milk, then set aside. Place the sugar into a pan along with 3 tbsp water. Over a gentle heat, cook without stirring for about 7 mins until the sugar melts and starts to turn golden brown. Add in the muesli, stir, then pour onto a tray lined with baking parchment paper. Leave to cool, then break into very small pieces.

Divide the chocolate mixture between the glasses and allow to cool, but don't refrigerate. Drizzle over the caramel crunch to serve.

Fudge Pie with Raspberries (12 Servings)

Per Serving = Calories: 294 – Fat: 23.4g – Carbs: 21.20g – Protein: 3.10g

Ingredients

- 50g raw cacao powder, plus extra to sprinkle
- 1/2 cup boiling water
- 1 cup caster sugar
- 150g coconut oil, melted, cooled
- 3 eggs, at room temperature
- 150g macadamia meal
- 1/2 teaspoon bicarbonate soda
- Pinch salt
- Raspberries, to serve
- Sprinkle of powdered sugar for garnish

Directions:

Preheat oven to 325F. Grease and line the base and sides of a springform pan with baking paper.

Combine cacao and boiling water in a small bowl. Stir quickly to blend the cacoa and water into a light syrup. Let the mixture cool slightly.

Using an electric mixer with the paddle attachment in a separate bowl, beat sugar, coconut oil and eggs for 3 minutes or until smooth and thickened.

Combine macadamia meal, bicarbonate and salt in a bowl.

With the mixer set on the low speed, beat the cacao mixture into the egg mixture. Add flour/powder mixture and stir until combined. Spoon batter into prepared pan and bake for 40-45 minutes or until a crust has formed on the top but the cake is still slightly wobbly. Stand pan on a wire rack for 10 minutes. Remove the sides of the pan and let it stand to cool completely. Remove the base of the pan.

Chill the cake before serving so that it will stay firm. Sprinkle with extra cacao and a touch of powdered sugar for contrast, and serve with berries.

Fudgy Rich Brownies (12 Servings)

Per Serving = Calories: 267 – Fat: 16g – Carbs: 33g – Protein: 2g

Ingredients:

- 250 grams (1 1/4 cups) granulated sugar
- 140 g (10 tbsp) unsalted butter
- 65 g (2/3 cup) Dutch process or "dark" cocoa powder
- 1 tsp instant espresso powder (optional)
- 1/2 tsp sea salt
- 1 tsp vanilla extract
- 2 cold large eggs
- 65 g (1/4 cup plus 2 1/2 tbsp) gluten free flour blend with no gums
- 125 to 140g (2/3 to 3/4 cup) dark chocolate chips/chunks

Directions:

Preheat oven to 350F. Line an 8 x 8-inch glass baking pan with parchment paper, leaving an overhang on 2 opposite sides.

In a large, microwave-safe bowl, combine the sugar, butter, cocoa, espresso powder (if using), and salt. Microwave in 20 to 30-second bursts, stirring after each time, until the butter is melted. Stir until everything is well mixed. Batter will be very grainy. Stir in the vanilla.

In this same bowl, add the eggs one at a time, stirring until combined after each one. Stir until the batter is thick and shiny. Add the flour and stir until thoroughly combined and no white streaks remain. Stir in chips or chocolate chunks and nuts if using. Spread evenly in the glass pan.

Bake until a toothpick comes out with a moist crumbs, 30 to 34 minutes. The top should be puffed and shiny and the brownies pulling away from the sides of the pan. Cool completely on a wire rack and then refrigerate. Cut into 12 for serving.

Lemon Coconut Cookies (14 Servings)

Per Serving = Calories: 100 – Fat: 4g – Carbs: 17g – Protein: 0g

Ingredients:

- 1 flax egg (1 tablespoon flax seeds + 3 tablespoon warm water)
- 4 tablespoons extra virgin coconut oil
- ½ cup sugar
- 1 teaspoon vanilla extract
- 2 tablespoon lemon juice
- 2 teaspoon lemon zest
- ½ cup rice flour
- ½ cup tapioca
- ½ teaspoon salt
- ½ cup shredded unsweetened dried coconut

Directions:

Preheat oven to 350 degrees °F and line a small cookie sheet with parchment paper.

Combine flax seeds and warm water to form an "egg," let sit for 5 minutes, then mix in a blender. Set to one side in a large bowl.

Beat coconut oil and sugar for about 5 minutes with a mixer in a separate bowl.

Mix flax egg, vanilla extract, lemon zest and juice in the flax bowl.

In a separate medium bowl, combine flour, tapioca and salt.

Add all of the dry ingredients to the wet ingredient, mix well to form a dough.

Add shredded coconut to the dough and stir until evenly moistened.

Spoon dough into a piping bag fitted with a piping tip. If the dough is very moist, chill in the fridge to set the dough.

Pipe the cookies onto the baking sheet, evenly spacing them.

Bake until golden, for 15-20 minutes.

Let the cookies cool on the tray for 10 minutes before eating or storing in an airtight container.

Pecan Sandies (22 Servings)

Per Serving = Calories: 125 – Fat: 7.5g – Carbs: 12.4g – Protein: 1.8g

Ingredients:

- 125g unsalted butter, softened
- 1/2 firmly packed cup (100g) brown sugar
- 1 large egg, lightly beaten
- 1 teaspoon vanilla extract
- 2 tablespoons natural yogurt
- 1 cup (150g) rice flour*
- 1 cup (150g) unsalted pecans with sultanas, roughly chopped

Directions:

Preheat the oven to 350F. Line 2 baking trays with parchment paper.

Using electric beaters, cream butter and sugar in a bowl until pale and thick. Add the egg and vanilla, and beat to combine.

Fold in yogurt, flour and nut mix with a flat rubber spatula. When the ingredients are thoroughly mixed, roll slightly rounded tablespoons of the mixture and place on the trays.

Flatten these cookies with either your floured fingers or a fork.

Bake in the oven for 12 minutes or until golden. Cool on the baking trays for 5 minutes, then transfer to a rack to cool.

Keep in an airtight container for up to 3 days.

Pumpkin Pie Filling (8 Servings)

Per Serving = Calories: 97– Fat: 2g – Carbs: 18g – Protein: 3g

Ingredients:

- 2 large eggs
- 1/2 cup granulated cane sugar
- 1 teaspoon ground cinnamon
- 1/2 teaspoon ground ginger
- 1/4 teaspoon ground cloves
- 1/4 teaspoon salt
- 1 - 15 oz. can pumpkin puree
- 1 cup unsweetened almond milk

Directions:

To make the filling, beat the eggs until frothy and yellow. Beat in sugar, cinnamon, ginger, cloves and salt, making sure the eggs and spices have no clumps. Add the pumpkin and milk and mix until the batter is smooth. Pour into a prepared pie crust.

Bake at 450 degrees F for 10 minutes. Reduce heat to 350 degrees F and bake for 50 to 60 minutes, or until middle is set.

Cool completely and chill. Serve with whipped cream (lactose free) and a sprinkle of nutmeg if desired.

Orange Cranberry Pudding (7 Servings)

Per Serving = Calories: 218– Fat: 6g – Carbs: 35g – Protein: 6g

Serving size ½ cup

Ingredients
- 1 cup orange juice
- 1½ cups fresh cranberries
- 1 cup quinoa, rinsed
- 2½ cups lactose-free milk
- ¼ cup maple syrup
- 2 teaspoons pure vanilla extract
- 1 teaspoon orange zest
- ½ cup sliced almonds, toasted

Directions:

Pre-heat oven to 400 degrees. Place cranberries and orange juice in a medium sauce pan, and heat until boiling. Reduce heat and simmer for approximately 5 minutes, or until cranberries have "popped" (this is always so fun!) and are cooked through.

Add quinoa, milk, maple syrup, vanilla, and orange zest to orange juice and cranberry mixture, and heat until boiling. Turn heat down to medium low and cover 2/3 of the pan. Cook pudding mixture for 30 minutes, or until pudding consistency is achieved. Continue to stir every 3-5 minutes to prevent the pudding from sticking. While quinoa is cooking, place sliced almonds on a baking sheet, and bake in oven for 4-5 minutes, or until lightly brown and toasted.

Divide quinoa pudding equally in to 7 serving dishes, and top with the toasted almonds. Serve warm, or chill the pudding in fridge, and serve cold.

Rhubarb Parfait (6 Servings)

Per Serving = Calories: 300– Fat:
20g – Carbs: 26g – Protein: 3g

Ingredients:

- 1 large bunch fresh rhubarb, cut into 2cm pieces
- 1/2 cup caster sugar
- 1 cup water
- 1 cup premium vanilla custard
- 300ml thickened cream, whipped (lactose free)

Directions:

Heat rhubarb, sugar and water in a saucepan over low heat, stirring so the sugar won't burn or stick. Cook, stirring, for 5 minutes or until sugar is dissolved. Bring to a boil.

Reduce heat and simmer for 20 to 25 minutes or until rhubarb is tender and mixture is thick. Set aside to cool to room temperature.

Gently fold custard and cream together but leave swirls of the light and darker color for effect. Layer custard mixture and rhubarb into crystal or clear serving glasses. Chill before serving.

Rice Pudding (4 Servings)

Per Serving = Calories: 547 – Fat: 9g
– Carbs: 104g – Protein: 11g

Ingredients:

- 1L (4 cups) milk
- 165g (3/4 cup) medium-grain rice
- 1/4 teaspoon salt
- 110g (1/2 cup) caster sugar
- 1 teaspoon vanilla extract
- Ground nutmeg for garnish

Directions:

Place the milk, rice and salt in a large saucepan over medium-high heat and bring to a boil. Reduce the heat to medium-low and cook, stirring, for 20 minutes or until the rice is tender.

Add the sugar and vanilla. Increase heat to medium-high and bring to a boil. Boil for 2 more minutes until the rice has softened and the mixture thickens.

Spoon the rice evenly among the four serving bowls. Sprinkle with nutmeg and a touch of cinnamon. Serve immediately.

Strawberries in the Clouds (4 Servings)

Per Serving = Calories: 394 – Fat: 22g – Carbs: 43g – Protein: 5g

Ingredients:

- 2 cups frozen strawberries
- 150ml thickened cream (lactose free)
- 100g packet meringue clouds
- 100g white chocolate, roughly chopped

Directions:

Place berries on a large plate lined with a paper towel. Stand at room temperature for 5 minutes to partially thaw.

Using an electric mixer, beat cream until soft peaks form. Using your fingers, gently crush the meringue nests (clouds). Add crushed meringue and white chocolate bits to the cream by gently folding to combine.

Transfer the fruit to a bowl. Gently mash the fruit with a fork. Slowly fold into the cream and meringue, barely stirring so as not to disturb the color. It adds more drama to the dessert if the color has not turned pink.

Spoon into four 3/4-cup capacity clear glasses. Cover. Refrigerate until ready to serve

Strawberry Crumble (4 Servings)

Per Serving = Calories: 728 – Fat: 31g – Carbs: 101g – Protein: 7g

Ingredients:

- 3/4 cup self-rising flour gluten free
- 1 teaspoon ground cardamom
- 125g butter, cubed, chilled
- 1/2 cup rolled oats
- 1 1/4 cup caster sugar
- 1/4 cup slivered almonds
- 1/2 cup water
- 500g frozen mixed berries, thawed

Directions:

Sift flour and cardamom into a bowl. Cut in the butter with a fork until the batter resembles breadcrumbs. Stir in rolled oats, 1/4 cup caster sugar and almonds. Cover and place in the fridge.

Preheat oven to 350F. Heat remaining sugar and water in a saucepan over medium heat. Cook, stirring, until sugar dissolves. Bring sugar water to a boil and then reduce the heat to low. Continue to simmer until the syrup reduces and thickens, about 7-10 minutes. Let the syrup cool.

Gently stir the berries into the cooled syrup. Spoon into 4 ramekins and sprinkle with the crumble batter that has been refrigerated.

Bake for 25 minutes or until golden, serve warm.

Conclusion

Thank you for purchasing this book, **Low FODMAP: 80 Easy and Delicious Gastrointestinal-Friendly Recipes to Comfort your Digestive Disorders.** I pray that you will find relief from your symptoms as you try the delectable recipes included in this book.

If you have found this content to be useful, please comment on Amazon.

I appreciate your comments.

Thank you,

Mary Criswell-Carpenter

www.marycriswellcarpenter.com

www.ingramcontent.com/pod-product-compliance
Lightning Source LLC
Chambersburg PA
CBHW060624290526
45793CB00001B/131